POWER HEALING – PRE-NATAL

FROM BEFORE TO AFTER BIRTH

PAUL ARDENNES

Copyright © 2015 and after by Univergy, LLC.

All Right Reserved.

I0420165

TABLE OF CONTENTS

INTRODUCTION

I wrote this book because pregnancy and birth are natural. Women should be working with them naturally to unleash their power.

A woman's body is designed for pregnancy and birth. It is instinctively prepared with the stamina, strength, and gift to nurture and encourage a natural pregnancy and birth. By supporting and sustaining its own intuitive and primal knowledge, medical intervention can be avoided and may become unnecessary.

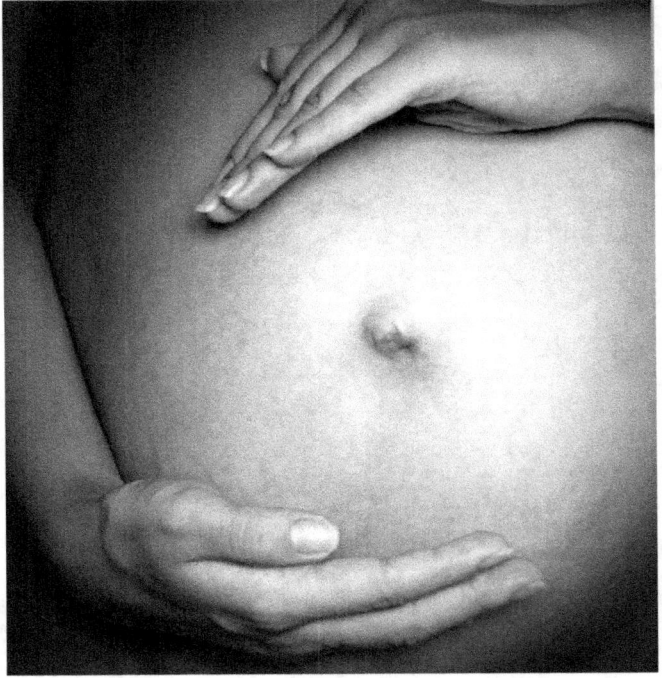

All over the world today, majority of women labor and give birth naturally, as they have since time immemorial. Natural pre-natal and natal care have been proven to be a nurturing, safe choice compared to hospital, doctor-assisted birth.

WHY YOU SHOULD READ THIS BOOK

This book will help you learn more about the natural methods for pregnancy and childbirth. It will teach you the external and internal positive elements and healthy environment that comprise natural pregnancy and birth. Here, you will know:

- The reasons why natural pregnancy and birth are important and the benefits that come with them.
- The proper natural pre-natal care practices.
- The importance of Neuromusicology in natural pre-natal care.
- The natural methods for childbirth and how to choose a suitable one for you.
- How to plan natural care practices for childbirth.

Though this ebook focuses on natural pre-natal and natal care, pre-conception care will be briefly discussed as well.

Happy reading!

CHAPTER 1. THE DISPLACEMENT OF NATURAL PRE-NATAL AND NATAL CARE

Conventional Western medicine is displacing the natural healing process of pregnancy and birth, stripping away its purpose and dignity. It made pregnancy a risky and perilous medical condition that needs to be cured and treated with increasing types and levels of technological and scientific interventions. What's worse, it took away the powerful, primal initiation that women need to go through towards motherhood. When the joy, delights, and bliss of giving birth are not experienced, a void is created, and eventually, its natural course is forgotten.

Pregnancy and birth are genetically encoded in women's bodies. Deviation from this natural order has inevitable consequences.

Conventional Western medicine is displacing the natural healing process of pregnancy and birth, stripping away its purpose and dignity.

Mothers today are unceremoniously thrown into the sacred sphere of motherhood with all the trauma and stress that comes with conventional birthing methods. Without the ecstasy of natural birth, women are observed to have an increasing level of depression and distress that were never seen before. As a result, babies experience more restlessness, colic, and reflux problems. Imprints have been made.

According to the World Health Organization, the statistics are saddening with depression and anxiety being diagnosed on children as young as four years old. Young people, too, especially those at the most important parts of their lives, are opting for diversions such as drugs, while others are committing suicide. We now live in a society where anxiety and depression are two of the major diseases seen worldwide. The effects of not acknowledging natural pregnancy and birth can be truly life-altering.

Thankfully, various health professionals from different research fields are looking at the birthing process to provide more benefits to the baby. Such step is challenging to achieve, considering many health professionals believe that pre-natal and natal care has no affect on babies. At this time and age, yes, many still think that way.

Dr. Raymond Castellino, a pioneer in the study of preventing and curing traumatic imprinting in babies, is developing a different kind of approach to pregnancy and birth. The approach is centered on the life of babies before and after birth, and is done with the family. Over time, imprinting within a baby affects family life, that's why such an environment is crucial. Therefore, it is now recognized that pregnancy and birth may have significant impact upon, and fundamental to, human development.

On one hand, empowering women or the babies separately is not going to provide any improvement in the displacement of pregnancy and birth. Imagine a competition between mother and baby, when there is none by nature.

CHAPTER 2. WHAT'S MISSING? NATURAL HEALING POWER

What's missing? Why is there displacement? Pregnancy and birth are suffering from a lack of these qualities that enable them to enjoy the natural process of healing:

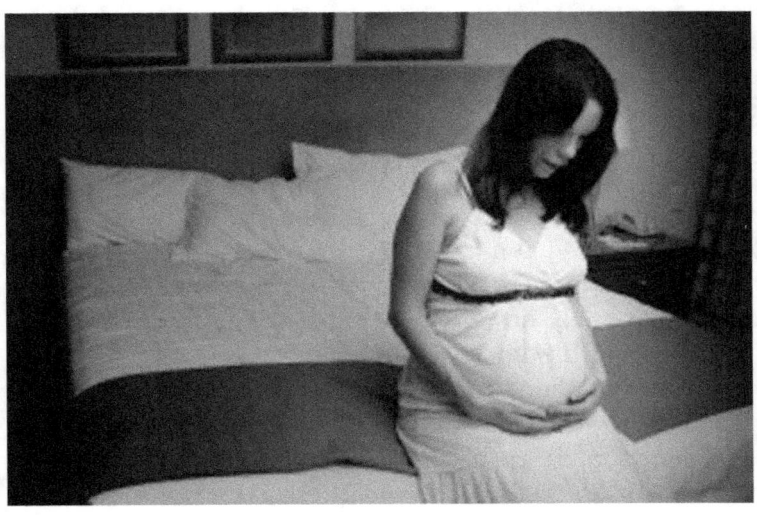

AUTHORITY AND CONTROL

It's easy to say that women have given excessive amounts of their authority and control to the medical system with regards to pregnancy and birth. A closer look needs to be done.

Science and Technology

The idea of power imbalance comes from a culture of putting faith in and prizing science and technological advancements. Rewards and unparalleled recognition are given to technology experts. Indeed, the world is better with their skills and inventions readily available to all. However, despite not wanting any technology involved in the birthing process, there are an increasing number of court cases against obstetricians for not using appropriate technology while delivering babies.

Information

Information is also something the world prizes today. In being pregnant and giving birth, a well-informed woman is considered responsible. However, having all the information is not the answer. The experience of giving birth cannot be supplied by mere information only. It must be felt firsthand. By relying on science, technology, and information, women disempower themselves. They diminish their own authority in pregnancy and birth by recognizing technology's hand as the sole power to help them in their condition. This creates an imbalance because naturally, a woman's body knows that it is made for motherhood.

Even the babies are providing information for mommies while still in their tummies. They are persistently informing their mothers of their desires and needs which lead mothers to intuitively feel how to best care for them. They do this through their placenta, which is a natural order of how babies and mothers communicate with each other during pregnancy (And perhaps a reason why Neuromusicology is beneficial, a topic to be discussed later in this ebook). In other words, it is a physiological (the study of the natural function of living things) truth.

Hormones, nutrients, and blood are constantly transferred and exchanged between mom and baby through the placenta. This in turn, instructs the mother's mind and body to provide the baby with specific mothering it needs and requires. Similarly, a mother's inclinations, dreams, yearnings, and cravings during pregnancy are felt and experienced by the baby as well. Such exchange of information between mother and child can never be explained or done by detailed, numerical information that medical tests and technology can do.

Speaking of medical tests, women can use the ancient system of intuition to determine if they are pregnant, instead of using a pregnancy test. The truth will eventually unfold itself, though gradually, but will allow women space to adapt and learn at their own pace, giving them a time to dream and reflect about what kind of pregnancy they want. If women choose to follow this traditional path, they are able to reinforce and discover an absolute power and unbreakable trust in themselves and in their bodies. Such power and trust is the best possible preparation method for pregnancy and birth. At the same time, it is based on responsibility because women are able to act based on the truth of their being. When this happens, it'll give women the choice to use medical opinion and care without losing their power.

Tapping into women's natural intuitions and primal instincts during pregnancy can open diverse communication channels with babies.

Furthermore, tapping into women's natural intuitions and primal instincts during pregnancy can open diverse communication channels with babies. This enhances psychic powers of communication that nature has assigned to mothers of all species. Being a mother can bring a woman to a state of deep thinking that satisfies both spiritual and emotional spheres – something that nature has purposely done from the beginning.

Wouldn't it be nice, if the society that humans live in accept that pregnancy and birth has its power? Wouldn't it be great to live in a world where technology is a tool, but not a master? Treatment of pre-natal and natal care would be different if that happens.

SUBMISSION

In popular culture, submission is not an accepted virtue. It is often viewed as a sign of weakness. Instead, women are told to become in control and active in their lives. Though true, the mere act of taking control is not always the perfect ingredient in all circumstances. Absolute force of will by itself for example, cannot help a woman give birth. A more subtle path of submission, but equally powerful, should be learned and undertaken.

The Female Body

Society today does not trust the natural order of things. This is evident on how modern women find it difficult to submit, because for them, it reflects a lack of confidence in their bodies. This thought is made even worse by the obstetric model enumerating exaggerated anomalies within the female body and suggesting numerous technological methods designed to "fix" them.

The Midwife

Women have also forgotten the guidance of a midwife in the birthing process. They are the patrons who, for centuries, have helped women through the transition to motherhood, where a thin veil between life and death is eternally present. Today, their services are still available to women. Their guidance is always ready to remind women that all the other women who gave birth before have passed their successful birth genes to women today. Therefore, women today also know how to give birth naturally with success.

The Female Ego

When women are consciously present while giving birth, they are allowing nature to take control by preventing rational mind to take hold. By doing so, women are able to access wisdom taught in spiritual traditions: that the female ego should not be a mistress, but rather a servant. When the female ego submits itself, the path to enlightenment and ecstasy is achieved. Through a woman's life of motherhood, this level of submission will also be helpful.

A profound experience for a woman giving birth is when deeper innate rhythms surface because of conscious submission. Eventually, a woman learns to be confident of the female body's natural rhythm while giving birth, as well that of the baby's. Such lesson is another of nature's gift that guarantees the maximum survival for babies and the best possible mothering women can provide.

Submission to natural pregnancy and birth also signifies women's role on earth: they are not the architects of creation, but life comes through them, gracefully and purely, when they allow it.

PASSION

All human lives began as a passionate act. All humans desire for the pleasure and intensity that is caused by the act of sex. In fact, many cultures believe that sexual act has the capacity for healing. Indeed, it is powerful. It gives humans the gift of creating a new life. At the same time, it offers a powerful experience where love, tenderness, excitement, pleasure, and hormone levels are at their peak. These experiences are also replicated during giving birth. In other words, the act of giving birth is also a sexual and passionate act. Hence, birth is the most passionate experience a woman can have just by looking at the hormone levels of both mother and baby during birth.

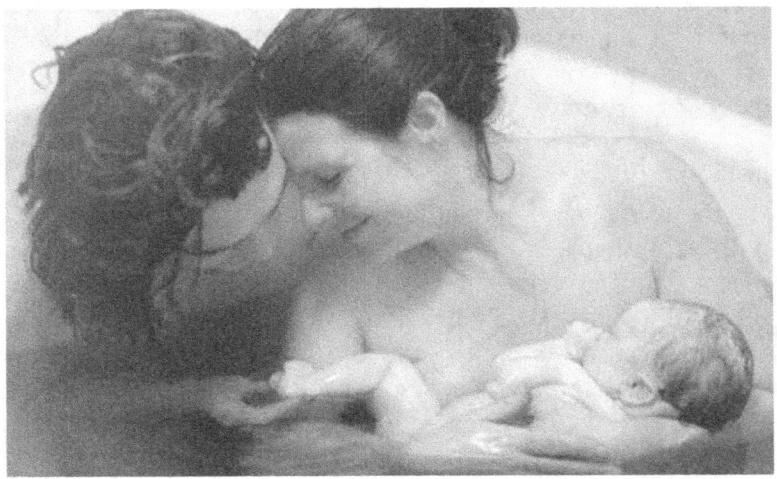

Hormone Levels

During labor, the hormone of love, otherwise known as Oxytocin, reaches its peak levels, releasing the most unselfish love between mom and baby. Hormones of transcendence and pleasure, also called Endorphins, are at their peak during birth. Noradrenaline (Norepinephrine) and Adrenaline (Epinephrine), the fight-or-flight hormones, are also present at their highest. The adrenaline and noradrenaline hormones cause excitement and amazement on both mother and baby at first contact. Such fight-or-flight hormones also prevent the baby from getting less oxygen during the final phase of birth. Meanwhile, the mothering hormone, Prolactin, helps women to yield to their babies. As a reward, it also gives women the utmost tenderness of maternal feelings.

Don't get these hormones wrong, however. They are not there just to make mother and child feel good. They are not just mere add-ons. Hormones actually coordinate sexual activity and the birthing process. They also enhance ease, safety, and efficiency of birth. Also, this cocktail of hormones rewards mothers with feelings of fulfillment and ecstasy, making them want to give birth repeatedly. In fact, all mammals share this experience at birth. It has even become a requirement for mothering in majority of species as it switches instinctive maternal behavior on.

Pain

On the other hand, having a passionate birth doesn't mean pain is not present, though this may happen to some mothers. As a huge life event, birth can be demanding physically and emotionally. However, pain can be bearable if a woman receives well-rounded support, and is confident with the female body. A woman can then respond based on instincts using the female body's own resources such as movement, sound, and breath – the most accessible and basic tools for giving birth.

Unfortunately, pregnancy and birth have become a medical affair, without passion and encouragement of emotional expression. The passion of birth is not acknowledged, or accommodated. To regain the passion of birth, women are to permit themselves to have a choice. They should choose their own birth attendants at a birth setting that they feel most comfortable in. With these circumstances, pregnancy and the birthing process will be easier.

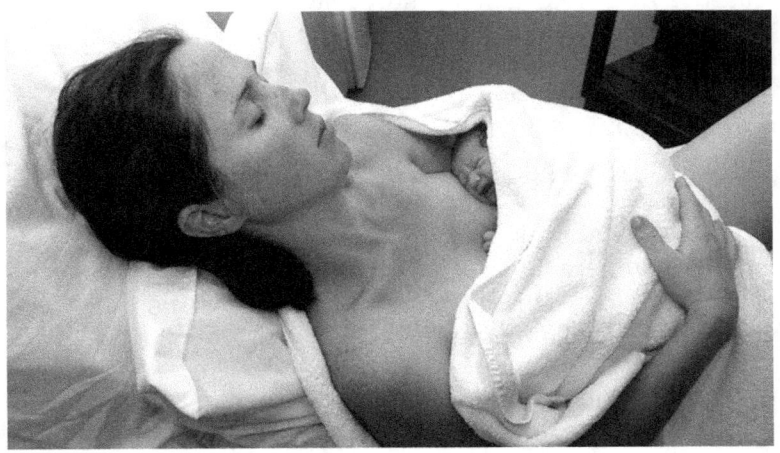

Healing Power

Passion has a healing power. It is an antidote and opposite for depression and despair, conditions imprinted in babies that were discussed in Chapter 1. This is true hormonally and physiologically. If women give birth and babies are born passionately, emotional imprints would be different, and better.

LOVE

Passion is powerful, but when combined with love, it becomes more so. Likewise, the two are powerful at birth and in the act of sex. As mentioned earlier, the hormone of love, Oxytocin, is released during birth. In sexual activity, the same thing happens. Again, hormones play a huge role in leading women towards ecstatic experiences. However, love, in the form of hormones, is extremely weak in the face of medical intervention. How can this happen?

During birth, the production of Oxytocin in a woman's body is significantly reduced. This is done with the use of pain relief and unfortunately, it prolongs labor. What's worse, by the time pain relief has worn off, a woman's body no longer has high levels of Oxytocin needed to give that last powerful contraction designed to give birth to a baby easily and quickly. As a result, it is more likely that forceps will be needed to pull out a baby from its mother. Sad, isn't it?

In another scenario, the drug Syntocinon (Pitocin), a synthetic form of Oxytocin, is also administered to a birthing mother. It is done so as to accelerate and induce labor. In many developed countries, many women receive large doses of this drug during birth. Although it helps, it can make mothers vulnerable to hemorrhage after giving birth and it also interferes with the body's Oxytocin system. The long-term effect is still unknown.

Women should claim and emphasize their innate power in pregnancy and birth. To do this, pregnancy and birth should be experienced the natural way. It should not be alienated to its natural order, unless humans want its powerful healing ability to stop. What is needed is the collective power, submission, passion, and love as women give birth to their babies.

Chapter 3. Benefits of Natural Pre-Natal Care

In the mid-20th century, women were encouraged to seek hospital care during childbirth. Obstetricians and other medical professionals organized birthing women based on their standards and studies. This led to the improvement of birthing practices. However, instead of favoring mother and baby, such practices only made it more difficult for them. As it turned out, certain birthing practices were only developed to favor medical professionals.

Preparing for a natural pregnancy and birth begins even before a woman becomes pregnant.

Soon after, natural pregnancy and birth were set in motion by various active birth movements. They were calling for the cut of medical intervention from pregnancy and childbirth. They wanted to focus on how mothers can empower themselves during their pregnancy and while they gave birth naturally.

Ideally, preparing for a natural pregnancy and birth begins even before a woman becomes pregnant. Women's good health helps babies become healthy, too. As a result, there are more choices in the birthing process where both mother and baby are healthy.

Start with Pre-Conception Care

To start a pregnancy in the most favorable health a woman could have, pre-conception care is important. Prior to conceiving, it intends to address the emotional and physical needs of a mother-to-be.

A pre-conception care visit or counseling can help women take the necessary steps for a healthy and safe pregnancy. It gives women the opportunity to learn an approach to their pregnancy and how to prepare for it. It typically covers:

- Choosing the best natural method for childbirth
- Knowing the best diet, exercise, nutrition, and supplementation to get pregnant
- Finding potential health problems such as toxin load, hormonal imbalance, diabetes, heart diseases or other medical conditions that can interfere with conceiving and healthy baby growth
- Addressing potential health complications
- Making sure a woman gets the necessary physical and emotional support for a healthy pregnancy

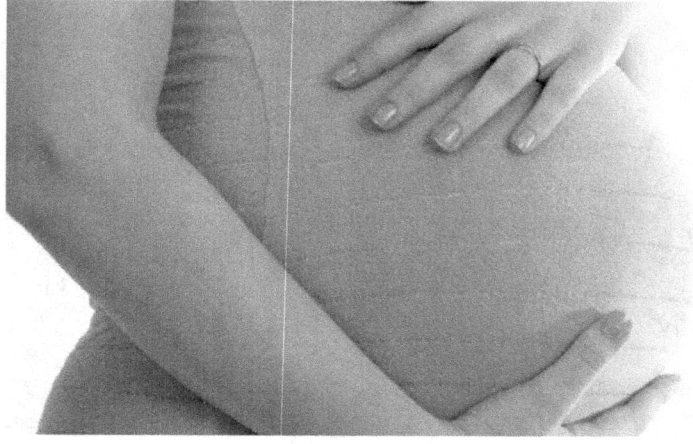

Before conception, there are a few months that serve as a window of opportunity for women to improve the quality of the actual conception itself, their pregnancy, and the health of their child. Certain lifestyle habits, diet, hormonal imbalances, and nutrient deficiencies can pose a threat to conception. Lack of support from experienced mothers and undiscovered pregnancy-related medical conditions are also big challenges to a woman. A natural approach to pre-conception and pregnancy can create a successful, healthy, and happy experience for both mother and baby.

Pre-conception care also discusses the birthing process, its risks, and spiritual values.

NATURAL PRE-NATAL CARE

Women pick out the baby's clothes and daydream about building a nursery room as soon as they learn they are pregnant. They are overjoyed and excited. As much as this is normal, preparing a woman's body for the wonderful and incredible journey is more important. One of the best things women can do to their soon-to-be babies is to get the best pre-natal care.

A natural approach to pre-natal care is important because conventional medicine is convinced that birth should be managed by modern medical practices. This idea proves that medical practitioners are not aware of the benefits of true natural birth, although they are sympathetic to the thought.

This idea is one of the reasons why there are stories of mothers who are disappointed of their birthing process. Because doctors have no idea of what a true natural birth is, they say yes to women who want an intervention and drug-free birth. Later on, they do exactly the opposite of what their patients asked for, thus leaving a devastating birthing experience.

A natural pregnancy care should be able to:

- Prepare a woman's body for birth
- Teach a woman how to get good sleep
- Help a woman create a birth plan
- Instruct a woman on the proper nutrition and exercise
- Prepare for a happy, fulfilling postpartum

Natural pre-natal care provides support in the following areas:

Emotional Inclination

Natural pre-natal care should be able to heal or clear out any grief or other depressing feelings cause by traumatic hospital birth experiences in the past.

Practitioner Evaluation

Pre-natal care helps women evaluate their chosen birthing practitioner. It is important for pregnant women to know if a practitioner is truly an advocate and is knowledgeable of natural birth. Pre-natal care is important, but the birthing process needs its expert guidance even more.

Information Validation

Usually, women who prefer a natural pregnancy are well-informed of their choices. They have done their research, but would want an expert to validate the information they've gathered. This could well be done by a midwife, doula, healthcare provider, or natural birth practitioner.

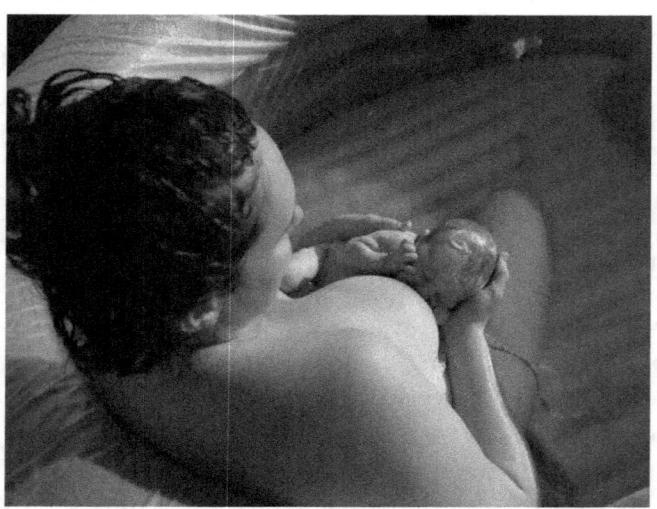

Breastfeeding Readiness

This is especially valuable for first-time moms. Natural pre-natal care should be able to prepare women to breastfeed their babies when there are no other experienced women to explain it to them.

A natural pregnancy should be provided with all these things. This is natural pre-natal care, but what are its benefits?

BENEFITS OF NATURAL PRE-NATAL CARE

Considers Women's Body, Mind, and Spirit
A natural pregnancy accepts the positive effects of a healthy mind and soul.

Natural pre-natal care includes the whole aspect of a woman, whereas in medical intervention, only the physical aspect is considered. Physical health, spirituality, emotional wellbeing, values and beliefs, and relationships, all shape pregnancy and birth.

A natural method includes body, mind, and spirit. In the physical aspect, proper nutrition and exercise are always discussed. Emotions and the mind are neglected most of the time when in truth, they also play a role in shaping the overall health of a pregnant woman. Beliefs and values are key to properly responding to support system, relationships, and stress.

The spiritual aspect on the other hand, is not exclusive to any specific religious beliefs. It's important to pregnancy care because it's that part of a woman that brings peace. It's a hard-to-explain aspect, but is crucial in the overall health of a mommy. Women should be able to determine which things, places, or time makes them feel calm and serene in order to have a peaceful pregnancy.

Uses Complementary and Alternative Medicine
A natural approach to pregnancy encourages use of complementary and alternative medicine (or CAM) and therapies to treat or prevent common complications and discomforts.

CAM is widely practiced today and is readily available for all. Despite this, many women still prefer conventional medications. Little do they know that majority of medications today aren't always safe for pregnant mothers. Massage and acupuncture, just to name a few, are good examples of alternative therapies that are considered safe for pregnant women. This prompts many medical practitioners, even doctors, to recommend extensive use of complementary and alternative medicine.

> *A natural approach to pregnancy recognizes the natural order of a woman's body: to conceive, nurture, and give birth.*

What's more, techniques used in CAM consider the physical, spiritual, emotional, and nutritional aspect of a woman's body, just like what's mentioned above. More importantly, with the help of natural therapies, meditation, massage, and herbs, it highlights the body's capacity for self-healing.

However, though it is encouraged, its application should be consistent with the mother's belief system. It should not be forced.

Trusts the Natural Order of Pregnancy and Birth

A natural approach to pregnancy recognizes the natural order of a woman's body. It strongly believes that a woman's body is naturally intended to conceive, nurture, and give birth. It changes to adapt to a baby's presence within the body.

Changes happen on the musculoskeletal, urinary, endocrine, cardiovascular, respiratory, and gastrointestinal systems. Changes also appear on almost on all parts of the woman's body including the abdomen, skin, and breasts. Temperature and body weight also changes drastically.

How can these benefits help women during their pregnancy?

A natural approach to pregnancy includes the overall being of a woman. It includes a support team that aims to acknowledge a woman's natural capabilities and enhance them. It promotes freedom of choice which maximizes a woman's potential to have the healthiest pregnancy possible. Lastly, it encourages the most natural succession of childbirth.

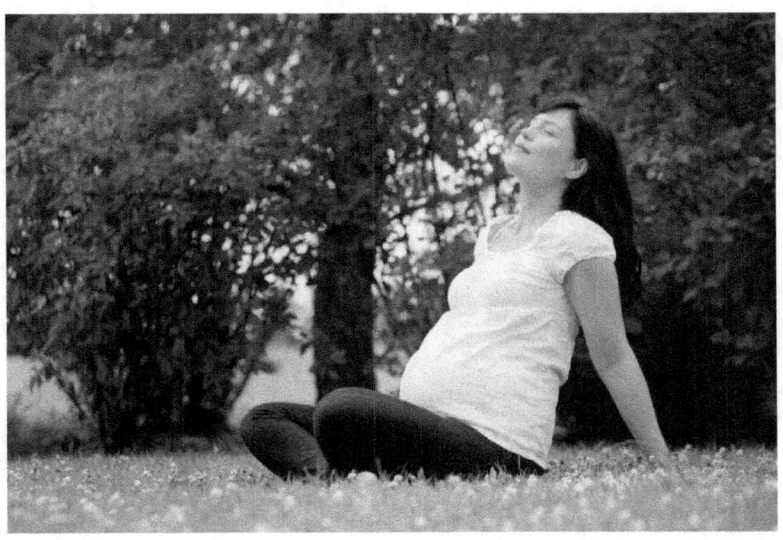

CHAPTER 4. NATURAL NATAL CARE

Many women today prefer a natural childbirth relying on techniques such as controlled breathing and relaxation to alleviate pain, instead of using medications. A natural childbirth puts a mother in control with the assistance of a natural labor practitioner offering gentle support and guidance throughout the stages of labor.

For soon-to-be mothers, many believe that being brave or becoming a martyr is not the main goal in natural childbirth. It's about treating childbirth as a perfectly natural event and experience. Women find it liberating, rewarding, and empowering.

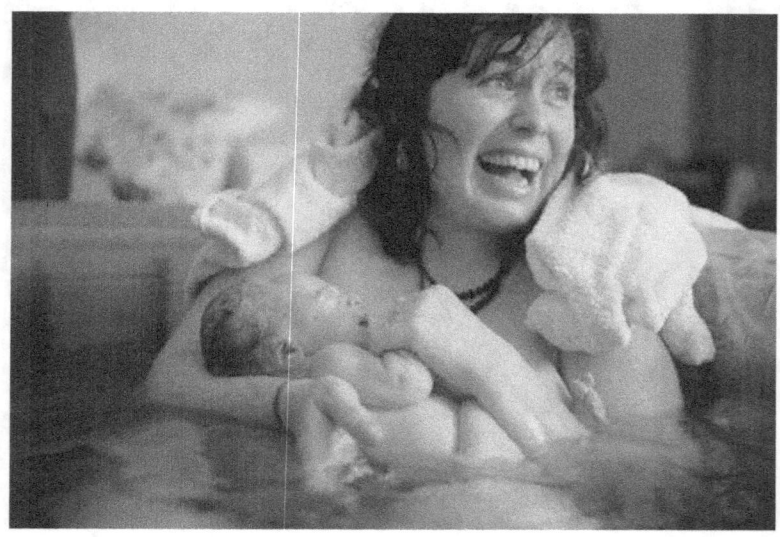

A natural childbirth means:

- Allowing women to take control of their labor and the delivery process in the most comfortable way possible
- Giving birth to a baby without using any medications especially pain relief
- Avoiding any kinds of medical interventions whenever or wherever necessary

Women who usually prefer natural childbirths are those with low-risk pregnancies. They want natural birth in order to avoid potential risks from drugs for the mother and baby, to have a better birthing experience, and to proactively deal with labor.

BENEFITS OF NATURAL CHILDBIRTH

Opting for a natural childbirth has its hidden benefits that most women are not aware of, such as:

Empowering

Natural childbirth makes women feel more confident and extremely empowered. Successfully getting through the tremendous demands of labor enables women to feel less fearful and stronger when tackling life's many other challenges. Hence, natural childbirth has always been described as powerful and mothers call themselves invincible.

Fulfilling

Women are fully conscious and alert when medications are not administered during labor. This makes them feel a deeper connection with their experience. There is a physical detachment when medications are given during childbirth because they dull women's senses. This leads to disappointment and sometimes, women are not even fully alert during their first contact with their baby, which is a crucial component of mother and baby relationship.

Liberating

Natural childbirth is liberating because it makes labor shorter. It takes away the pain of labor faster. Medications for pain often lead to longer contraction intervals and delivery because they interfere with how the female body naturally deals with labor. Sometimes, when intervals between contractions are prolonged, there's a tendency that women may not feel contractions at all. This is crucial because contractions tell women when to push. Without that order, women miss the natural rhythm of their body during labor.

> *Women who give birth naturally can feel better quickly after delivering babies.*

Safer and Healthier

Pain relief during labor often leads to more medical interventions. Epidurals for example, cut women off from the natural action of childbirth, reducing normal pushing and prolonging labor. This leads to doctor's intervention and when a medical professional is involved, synthetic Oxytocin may be administered. This has been mentioned in Chapter 1. It induces labor and causes hemorrhaging. It also increases risks of fever to develop on the mother which may lead to use of antibiotics. Forceps or a vacuum may also be used to pull the baby out of the birth canal. A fetal monitor may also be used to track the baby's heart rate. There's a likelihood that any of these may happen if Epidural or medical pain relief is used.

Makes Breastfeeding Easy

Babies born naturally show more interest in breastfeeding. The reason could be behind the use of pain relief, again. It interferes with the babies' instinct to suckle normally. In fact, with Epidural use, babies come out seemingly "drugged" and as a result, they find it difficult to latch on and, their suck and swallow behavior is uncoordinated which could last for hours an sometimes, even days.

Faster Healing Time

When there are no needles, tubes, or numbing drugs are used during childbirth, women who give birth naturally can feel better quickly after delivering babies. As soon as giving birth, naturally birthing mothers can walk around or do simple tasks. This is because of the release of the female body's Endorphins, hormones that relieve pain and have a calming effect. When a birthing mother is given Epidural during childbirth, release of Endorphin is reduced.

It's a good thing that in recent years, there has been a rise in women wanting to give birth naturally. Women who embrace this concept view childbirth as an extension of their lives. With many natural labor advocates and practitioners available today, women are finally receiving the support they need to have a natural birth. Women should always be respected for their choices.

Chapter 5. Natural Pre-Natal Care Practices

A healthy pregnancy doesn't happen on its own. Sometimes, unavoidable things happen, and other times, there are medical conditions that affect pregnancy. However, steps can be taken to make sure that a woman will have a natural, healthy pregnancy. This chapter outlines the steps women can take and choices they can make as their pregnancy progresses.

Bad and Good Habits

It is a general rule for pregnant women to live with their usual lifestyles, but do so in moderation. Here are bad habits to avoid and good habits to keep during pregnancy:

Bad Habits to Avoid

A pregnant woman needs to give up the following bad habits:

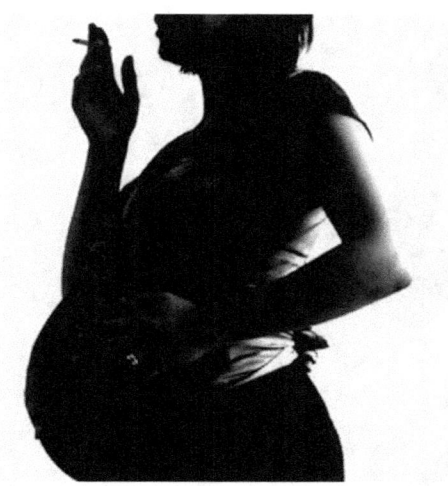

Smoking

Smoking is the worst habit any pregnant woman can have. It reduces the required quantity of oxygen that should reach the baby. Women should know that when a baby lacks oxygen, it can lead to a weak heart and lung infections.

What's worse, it may even cause stillbirth or miscarriages. It also affects the body's blood circulation.

In any case a woman feels like smoking even when pregnant, no alternative, vaping, or any form of patches can offer a less damaging effect. Indeed, smoking should be stopped immediately.

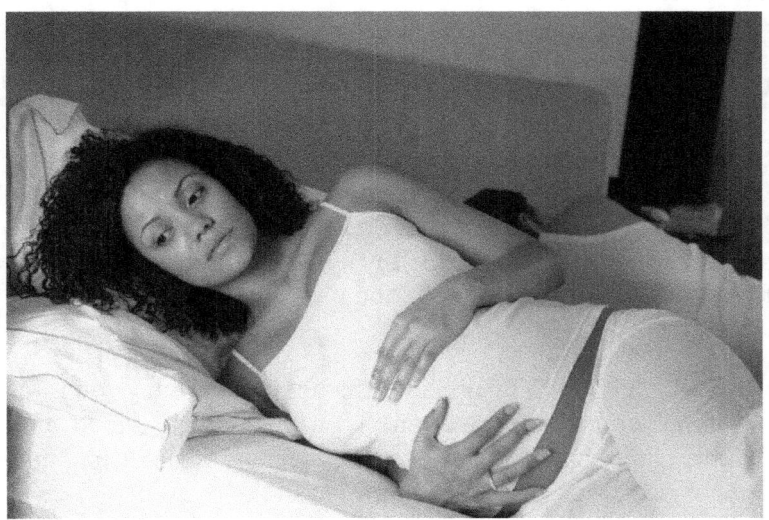

Lack of Sleep

According to a study from the University of Washington, pregnant women who sleep less than six hours a day during the first trimester have increased chances of Preeclampsia and high blood pressure.

Caffeine Intake

Too much caffeine in a pregnant woman's diet can increase risk of low birth weight for the baby, or worse, miscarriage. At the same time, it acts as a diuretic, which means it expels water from the body at increased amounts. As it does this, it also washes away important nutrients even before the body gets to absorb them.

Other sources of caffeine include pain killers, energy drinks, chocolate, colas, and tea. The allowed maximum amount of caffeine for a pregnant woman is 200mg per day. However, it is suggested for women to totally stop caffeine intake when pregnant.

> *Bad habits can harm both the mother and baby, often resulting to brain damage, growth issues, and diseases.*

Eating Junk Food

Pregnant women have unusual food cravings during the first three months of pregnancy. This occurs anytime of the day. Sometimes, junk food is in the list of foods they crave for. Unfortunately, junk food is not healthy for pregnant women. It has high levels of sugar and fats which are known to cause several birth defects. Unhealthy junk food can also lead to high sugar, cholesterol, and blood pressure levels.

Drugs and Alcohol

Without question, drugs and alcohol are dangerous for pregnant women. Drugs of any type, unless prescribed by a doctor, is outright dangerous. Alcohol meanwhile, can cause serious problems in the development of the baby.

These bad habits can harm both the mother and baby, often resulting to brain damage, growth issues, and diseases. For a healthy pregnancy and baby, keep off these habits.

Good Habits to Keep

These are the good habits a pregnant woman should keep:

Sleep More

Pregnant women feel extra sleepy all the time and this is perfectly normal. It is most likely to happen only in the first trimester. When the urge to sleep occurs within anytime of the day, pregnant women should listen to their bodies and take a nap when needed. Taking occasional naps and resting makes a pregnant woman feel rejuvenated and energized. Also, this is one of the reasons as well, why caffeine intake should be avoided or reduced.

Moving Around

Exercise during pregnancy prevents excessive weight which could prove to be harmful to the overall health of both baby and mother. It also prevents gestational diabetes. More importantly, it sets the body to a fitness level that will help in childbearing and childbirth. However, pregnant women should never overdo workouts. Take simple walks, swimming, yoga, or jogging (More on this topic on a separate section later in this chapter).

Healthy Eating and Drinking

Pregnant women should get into the habit of eating healthy, especially during snack time. Nutritious snacks should always be kept within reach in case cravings occur. Healthy snacks include whole-grain crackers, yogurt, trail mix, granola, cheese sticks, dried or fresh fruits, and nuts. Pregnant women should also keep themselves hydrated. Water or fruit juices are the best choices.

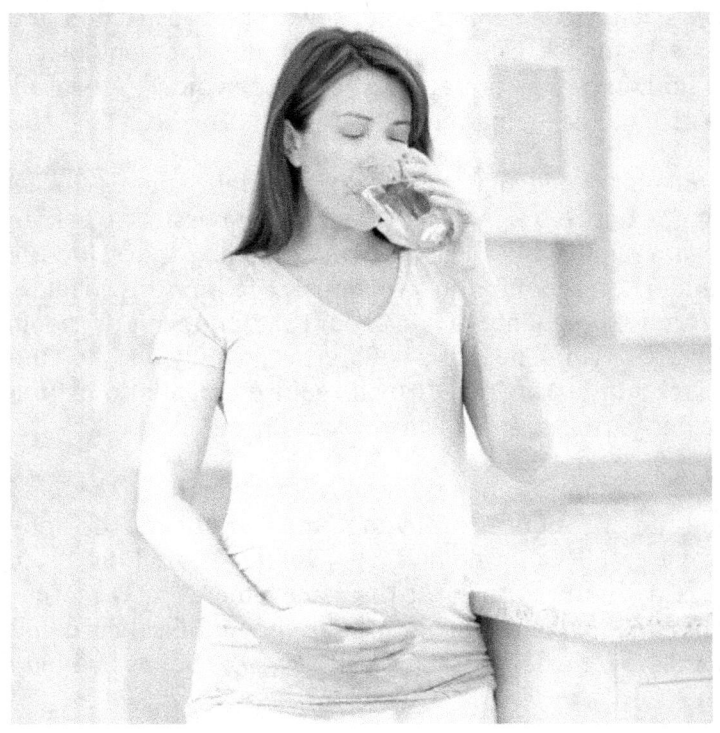

It is important for pregnant women to stay relaxed all the time. Studies have proven that increased level of stress leaves an imprint on the baby and leads to depression and anxiety later in life. Find a technique for relaxation and stick to it.

WEIGHT AND DIET

Certain muscles, the breasts, and the uterus increase in size during pregnancy. Aside from these, the increasing amniotic fluid, expanding membranes, enlarging placenta, and growing fetus all contribute to a pregnant woman's weight gain. However, the amount of exercise and food intake affects health and weight. Body parts may expand and increase in size, but only diet and exercise can determine how healthy a pregnant woman's weight is. If there is too much weight gain, childbirth will most likely be difficult because the baby could be oversized. On the other hand, severe diet restriction and excessive exercise can disrupt proper development of the baby. Both extremes therefore, should be avoided. A healthy weight should be maintained.

It is recommended that a pregnant woman gain 22-26 lbs during the entire pregnancy period. For the first 12 weeks, a little gain should be observed, while gaining more for the remainder of the months. Obviously, to do this, diet is important. A pregnant woman should eat food with nutrients enough for two. The baby will grow rapidly in the 2nd trimester and by this time, it will require essential nutrition particularly iron, calcium, vitamins, and protein.

Also, a pregnant woman's blood volume starts to expand around the 2nd month and by the time birth nears, the body will have 50-60% more blood. This volume is vital for a safe and healthy natural birth. At the same time, what a mother eats is absorbed by the baby through the umbilical cord and placenta. Now the food that the baby absorbs builds its blood supply.

For pregnant women, daily dietary items should include the following food groups: (1) healthy oils and fats, (2) dairy products, (3) citrus and other fruits, (4) yellow vegetables, (5) leafy green vegetables, (6) whole-grain products, and (7) protein foods.

HERBALS AND NATURAL SUPPLEMENTS

Miscarriage, cleft palate, pre-eclampsia, Gestational Diabetes, defects in vital organs, Cystic Fibrosis, Scoliosis, deafness, Hypoplasia, and Spina Bifida, are all associated with vitamins and mineral deficiencies. They can all be prevented by a good natural pregnancy regimen. Here is a list of a few of natural supplements a pregnant mother should take:

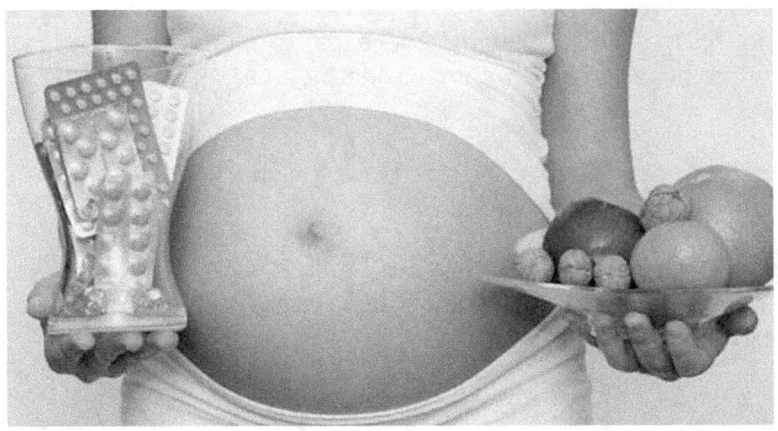

Fermented Cod Liver Oil or an Omega 3 supplement
Omega 3 has many benefits for pregnancy. It is known to help visual and neurological development in the baby. After birth, it is essential in helping mothers produce breast milk. At higher doses, it helps increase birth weight of babies, reduces allergies in babies and depression in mothers, prevents premature labor and delivery, and lowers risk of Preeclampsia. Aside from cod fish, other excellent sources of Omega 3 are herring, anchovies, tuna, salmon, and sardines.

Rosehip or Vitamin C Chewable

Take 2–4/day to lower baby's risk of infection, speed up natural healing, reduce labor, toughen the perineum, reduce hemorrhoids and varicose veins, and of course, provide daily dose of vitamin C.

Red Raspberry

Take 2-3/day to facilitate a healthy pregnancy, birth, delivery, and recovery. It also strengthens the uterus.

Methyl Folate

Take once a day to prevent birth defects including incomplete development of the spinal vertebrae or cord (Spina Bifida). It also prevents Anencephaly, or the underdevelopment of major parts of the brain. Alternative sources of Folic Acid include eggs, cantaloupe, asparagus, white beans, broccoli, spinach, lentils, and fortified cereals.

Zinc

Take once a day to prevent Down's Syndrome, cleft palate, clubbed limbs, Spina Bifida, etc.

B-vitamin Complex

Take twice a day to develop and support the digestive and nervous systems.

Herbal Trace Minerals

Take 2-3/day. It promotes healthy development of the baby by providing needed highly absorbable minerals.

Herbal Calcium, and Vitamin A and D

Take 2-3/day. It prevents poor bone formation, deafness, and birth defects.

Hawthorne

Take 2-3/day for healthy and proper development of the baby's heart.

Gotu Kola

Take 2/day, one in mid-morning and 1 in the evening. It decreases cellulite formation during pregnancy. It also aids in the baby's proper brain development.

Magnesium Complex
Take twice a day for bowel regularity and nervous system development.

Vitamin E with Selenium
Take once a day to help prevent genetic disorders, infant death, poor birth weight, Cystic Fibrosis, and Scoliosis.

Chromium
Take once a day to reduce the risk of gestational diabetes in pregnant women.

Wild Yam
Take 2/day for the first trimester to prevent miscarriages.

Chelated iron or yellow dock
To be taken for prevention of anemia.

Protein Shake
To be taken by pregnant vegetarian women for extra protein.

Probiotics
To be taken to alleviate pregnancy discomforts such as diarrhea and constipation.

Remember, these supplements do not work as substitutes. They are to complement a pregnant women's diet regimen.

EXERCISES

Exercise during pregnancy is important. It helps increase blood volume. It also increases endurance and stamina that a pregnant woman needs for labor. It also provides the baby with plenty of oxygen. Best of all, it helps pregnant women feel good about themselves. Here are some of the best physical activities for pregnant women.

Pre-Natal Belly Dancing

Belly dancing for pregnant women is a much loved exercise of many. Not only it helps them love their pregnant form, it also gets the heart pumping, which makes it good for the cardiovascular system of both mom and baby.

Walking

Walking is the most basic exercise, which makes it easy for pregnant women to do it. It causes a ripple effect by first, keeping the pelvis aligned; second, the baby responds by lining up properly; third, provides an easy labor. Three to five miles of walk, at a simple and easy pace, a day can be beneficial. It can also be broken into a few miles each walk, as long as the required miles are filled up.

Resistance Workouts

Resistance workout is also good for pregnant women. This is true for those who were into resistance workout routines before they were pregnant. Their bodies already know the intensity. Good options include pregnancy-safe kettlebell routines and resistance bands. Pregnant women are only allowed an intensity workout of five to eight.

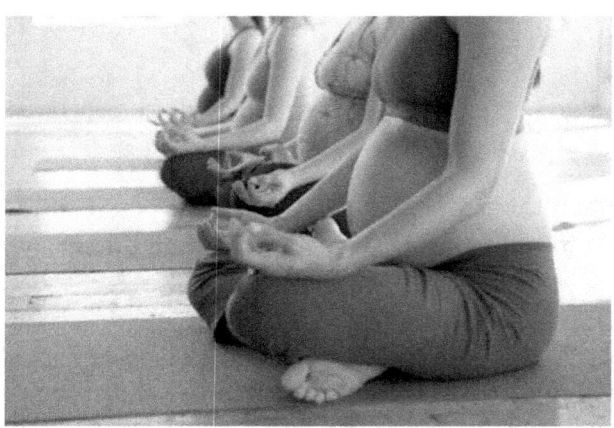

Pre-Natal Yoga

Another soothing routine, done daily or weekly, for pregnant moms is pre-natal yoga. It promotes two important skills for childbirth: breathing and squatting. It also reduces anxiety and stress, and improves sleep. It also lessens headaches, nausea, symptoms of carpal tunnel syndrome, and lower back pain. It also increases endurance, strength, and flexibility of muscles needed for the birthing process.

On the whole, the best exercise advice for pregnant women is for them to do what their bodies tell them to do. In other words, don't overdo exercise.

MENTAL ATTITUDES

During pregnancy, women feel a wide range of emotions: excitement, happiness, sadness, apprehension, shock, awe, joy and a whole lot of other feelings. Most of the time, they are easy to manage. Other times, they are stressful to deal with, which leads to pre-natal depression, even with the most joyous start.

Pregnant women should have all the support they need from their family and friends. At the same time, getting enough sleep, making time for walking, eating well, and taking care of themselves physically can help battle depression and anxiety. To enjoy the joy of pregnancy more, here are some tips for pregnant moms:

- Take birthing classes. It helps pregnant women to: empower themselves, understand how to work with their bodies, and make smart choices. It also helps them to work and bond with their babies to ensure a safe natural birth. Being in a class also opens up opportunity to talk with other pregnant women and share experiences with each other.
- Bond with the baby. Talk, write, or read a book to them. Shopping for baby items can also be relaxing. Pregnant women can do anything that can form a connection between them and their babies. Listening to music together can also form bonds.
- Stick to relaxing physical activities such as walking daily, yoga or any prenatal exercise.

- Spend time outdoors. Nothing beats a refreshing scenery to the mind. It clears off any worries or feelings of sadness.

Pre-Natal EFT

EFT is Emotional Freedom Technique. It is a powerful, life-altering tool used to gently and effectively release deep-rooted fears about giving birth. Healing professionals use it to make sure pregnant women are feeling emotionally stable when they go through the birthing process. Its techniques include the following:

- Provide a stress-free and comfortable birthing process and environment.
- Transform a mindset of fear into real excitement.
- Clear trauma imprinted on pregnant women from when they were born in order to avoid the same trauma from repeating again on their own birthing process.
- Set the mind to do and say what it wants and needs in order to create a desired childbirth outcome.
- Identify unique fears about childbirth and clear them permanently.

DRESSING – MATERNITY CLOTHES

Dressing can be a major fashion challenge for pregnant women. During pregnancy, the female body constantly changes, that's why it's not easy to choose the right clothes. However, choosing the right clothes makes pregnant women feel good about themselves thus, preventing depression and providing a satisfying experience. Here are the do's and don'ts of dressing for pregnant women:

Embrace That Baby Bump

Pregnant women should not be scared or embarrassed to show their baby bump. Instead, they should wear maternity clothes that fit well. Some women wear bigger non-maternity clothes to hide their bump, but actually make them look bigger.

Wear Some Color
Typically, pregnant women wear dark-colored clothes to make them look thinner. Actually, adding color to clothes flatters the body.

Wear Comfortable Jeans
Skinny jeans are in trend nowadays. However, pregnant women can still wear a good pair of jeans, as long as it makes them comfortable. Also, jeans can be paired with any type of clothes.

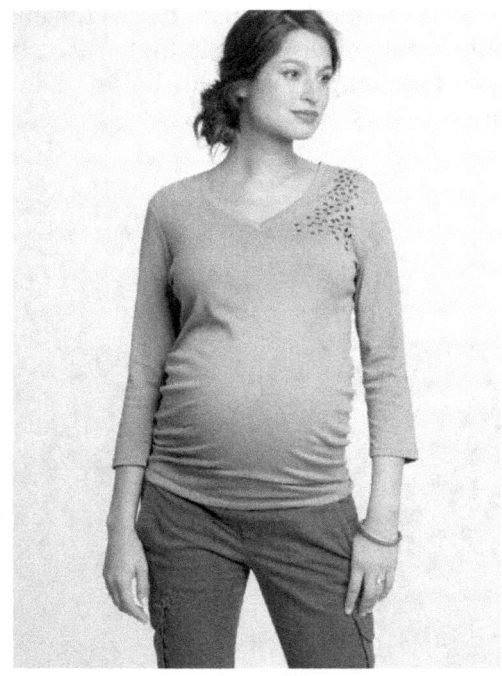

Layer Clothes Properly
Layering clothes can only look good on pregnant women if done properly. Otherwise, it'll make them look bigger. The rule is to layer clothes based on the body proportion.

Wear Stripes and Patterns

Pregnant women are often scared to wear clothes with stripes or patterns. Little do they know that patterns and stripes actually flatter the baby bump. Pregnant women should opt for all-over patterns or prints, and simple stripes.

Avoid Wearing Oversized Sweats

The most important thing when choosing the right maternity clothes is comfort. Although sweatpants and sweatshirts are comfortable to wear, they are not the only available options for pregnant women. Try leggings, dresses, and jersey knits.

MUSIC AND THE BABY – NEUROMUSICOLOGY

Music is beneficial both to mother and baby during pregnancy. For pregnant moms, music can help them relax. It controls their anxiety. More importantly, it helps them achieve an overall emotional-physical well-being.

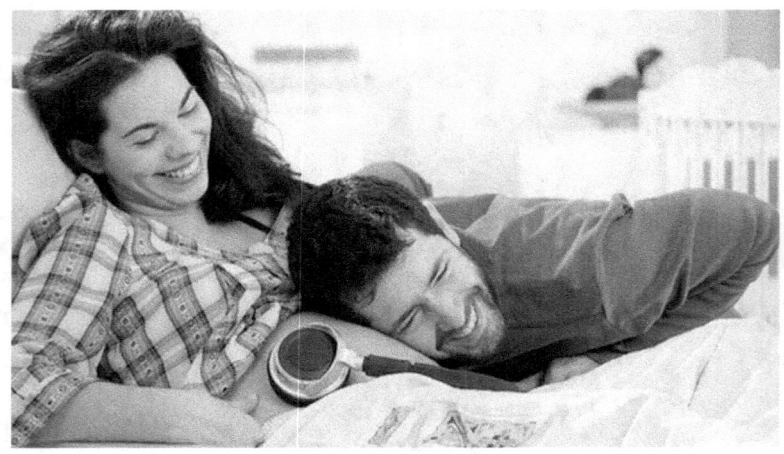

Music for the Mother

Pregnancy brings with itself various physical and emotional discomforts. Music has the ability to improve a pregnant woman's physical and emotional health. Pre-natal music therapy sessions provide a way on how mothers-to-be can prepare for the birthing process. A session includes pregnant women listening to music, their own voices, and internal rhythms as they respond to motor actions and changes in their bodies as pregnancy progress. By studying musical activities of pregnant women, techniques are learned on how to provide a better pregnancy and childbirth experience for women. This allows pregnant women to respond to the natural signs given to them by their bodies and babies.

Music for the Baby

Music therapies also stimulate the baby and encourage bonding between mom and baby. During pregnancy, music serves as a communication channel for mother and child, allowing mothers to create a serene and balanced emotional relationship with their babies. It also improves the growth of their baby's nervous system by stimulating its functional and structural development. All stimulation, external and internal sounds, during the baby's growth contribute to the development of the acoustic and sensor pathways in them. Based on studies, babies like the sound of voices of their mothers including its melody and tone. Both these elements act as channels of emotions from the mother to the baby. It acts as a cuddle of sound to the baby and informs them that their mother is excited to see them.

Listening to Positive Music

Listening to positive music is relaxing and soothing. For pregnant women, it encourages anxiety control, and creates pleasant and positive images. Slow, calm, and sweet music and genre bring to mind scenes from childhood and natural places. During labor, these images are then brought to mind between contractions, which distracts women and enable them to renew and regain strength, getting ready for the next big push. Listening to positive music is also used during the first stages of childbirth.

Singing during Pregnancy

Singing not only helps pregnant women improve their breathing, it also contributes to the healthy development of their babies. Studies about EVP, or electronic voice phenomena, show that a voice, either coming from a mother or father, stimulates the baby inside the womb. In fact, findings include stronger upper body in babies of professional female singers who sang while they were pregnant. Professional male singers on the other hand, had babies who walked at an early age.

Pre-natal singing also promotes healing. Endorphins are released when pregnant women sing. As a result, it reduces perception of pain, relaxes breathing, and produces fewer contractions.

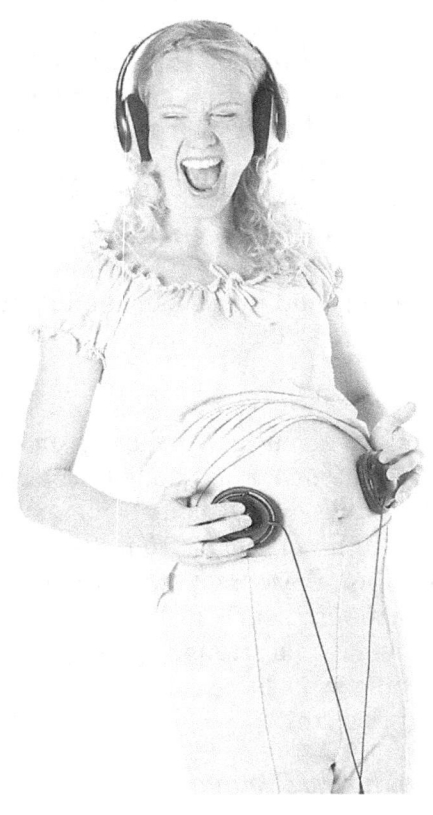

CHAPTER 6: NATURAL NATAL CARE PRACTICES

How can women be prepared for a successful and healthy natural birth? Are there more ways to prepare, or is natural childbirth just a matter of trusting the female body? What happens to a woman's body during labor and childbirth?

Getting ready for childbirth is one of the most important aspects of preparing for the arrival of the baby. Here is how to prepare for a natural childbirth:

WHAT TO DO FIRST

Natural birth begins even before the first signs of labor are felt. Major preparation is needed. Like athletes, pregnant women need to train physically and mentally. However, training doesn't have to be intense. They simply have to condition themselves positively by enrolling in birth classes, reading natural childbirth stories, and watching videos of natural deliveries.

Pregnant women also need to learn birth skills, positions for labor, and relaxation techniques. Practicing relaxation techniques, visualizing what women want for example, is an excellent method of natural birth preparation.

Pregnant women should also find and listen to good birth stories. Knowing about the experiences of other women is empowering and inspiring. How to use tools for labor should also be learned. This could sometimes be taught by childbirth professionals.

BE INFORMED

Information about the birthing process has been useful in helping women achieve more success with natural birth. There are pre-natal classes where women can learn more about pregnancy, birth, and baby care. Books and websites are also good sources of information.

Another excellent way to prepare is to gather all the support a pregnant woman can get. Doing this benefits both mom and baby, and dad, too.

TESTS

There are various tests and procedures that are needed during pregnancy and birth. Fortunately not all of them require doctor's intervention. A midwife or certified childbirth professional can administer them. Remember, each option should be carefully researched before consenting to any of them.

First Visit Blood Tests and Pap Smear

Though unnecessary, this it to ensure that a pregnant woman is not anemic during pregnancy and that there is no STD present. Women who regularly monitor their Vitamin D and blood levels may opt out from this test. However, after-birth routines may be done if that is the case. Also, these tests can reveal RH problems.

Remember, each test should be carefully researched before consenting to any of them.

Ultrasounds

Ultrasound is used to diagnose various aspects of a baby inside the womb including size and gender. However, there is some debate about its necessity and safety. In non-high risk cases, ultrasound may not be needed unless there is a specific risk.. A mother should carefully research and weigh this option. Qualified midwives and childbirth professionals can feel the position, size, and movement of the baby without using ultrasounds.

Fetal Dopplers for Heartbeat

Dopplers are the instrument used to listen to the baby's heartbeat. However, there are issues with their use which makes doctors avoid using them for worry of passing on some radiation to the baby. Many midwives and childbirth professionals avoid using them, too. A fetoscope may be used as an alternative.

Urine Tests

Urine test is non-invasive and important because it reveals ketones or sugars in the urine which signifies health problems associated with headache, rapid weight gain, and blood pressure changes.

Blood Pressure Checks

Also non-invasive, this test determines high-blood pressure which is dangerous for pregnant women especially when there is preeclampsia involved.

Internal Exams

Though popular, internal exams are unnecessary. An internal exam such as a cervix check is done to see how far dilated a woman in labor is. This is inaccurate and creates a chance for bacteria to enter the vaginal area.

Glucose Test

A Glucose test is done to check for gestational diabetes. They are only recommended for women with history of diabetes in their family or for lifestyle reasons. Otherwise, it is unnecessary.

Group B Strep

This test is done to check if pregnant women have Group B Strep or GBS, a life-threatening infection. A baby is at risk of acquiring it at birth from an infected mother. The usual treatment is antibiotics. However, it is important to note that GBS screening is somewhat controversial and that antibiotics have bad effects on babies. The best thing to do is to treat it naturally with lots of Probiotics.

Kick Counts

Kick counts is a non-invasive way of checking if the baby is moving less inside the womb especially in the 3rd trimester of pregnancy. Fetal movement is important within a 2-hour stretch. If no movement is felt within this period, the baby could be in distress and needs immediate medical care.

Optional Screenings during Pregnancy
There are other optional screenings that can be done during pregnancy.

- First-trimester and maternal blood screening – to see if baby is at risk of birth and heart defects
- Amniocentesis (also called amnio) – to see if the baby has a genetic by testing the amniotic fluid around it
- Chorionic villus sampling (CVS) – to see if baby has a genetic condition.
- Cystic fibrosis carrier screening – to see if a pregnant woman has the gene that causes the Cystic fibrosis disease, which can be passed on to the baby. It affects digestion and breathing.

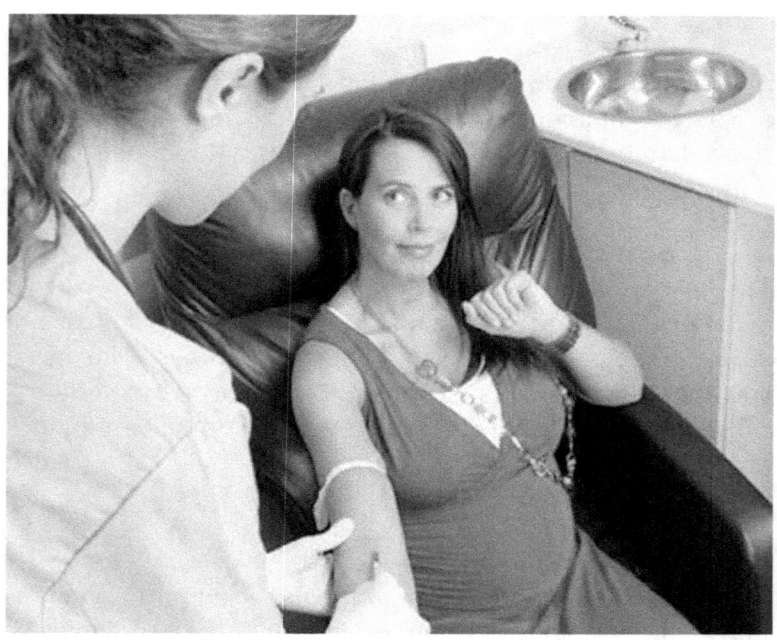

CHAPTER 7: NATURAL BIRTH METHODS

HISTORY

In modern history, natural birth reemerged as a popular method of childbirth during the 1950s and 1960s. Women were increasingly becoming aware of the complications brought about by the use of anesthesia during labor. They were noticing the bad side effects not only on women, but in babies as well. Not able to do anything about it, they started to demand control over their births. Finally, control shifted from the physicians to the women and their midwives. The natural childbirth movement and advocacy was born. There was an intense opinion that women should be in control of the childbirth experience, not their healthcare provider.

Eventually, advances in non-medicinal pain relief methods were discovered and made. Early advocates of natural childbirth include Lamaze, Bradley, Dick-Read, and Leboyer. They developed methods to prepare women for childbirth that included water immersion, hypnosis, patterned breathing, and relaxation. Women then began to repossess their independence in the birthing process when they were encouraged by the methods introduced by these early experts.

TYPES OF NATURAL BIRTH METHODS

When choosing a natural option, without any medical intervention, for giving birth, there are a number of different techniques that women can choose from. The following methods have been successfully used for many years in making natural birth a dream come true for many women. For natural birth candidates, it is important to take time to study these methods and identify which might work best. It is highly recommended to talk to a midwife or childbirth professional about different options.

Homebirth

Giving birth at home has been done in many countries all throughout history. Various cultures worldwide view birth as a vital part of family life. Today, majority of women still prefer to do so at home, or in a non-hospital setting. Today, a successful and safe homebirth can be achieved if it is carefully monitored. Another factor that can affect it is, if pregnant women are given proper care during pregnancy.

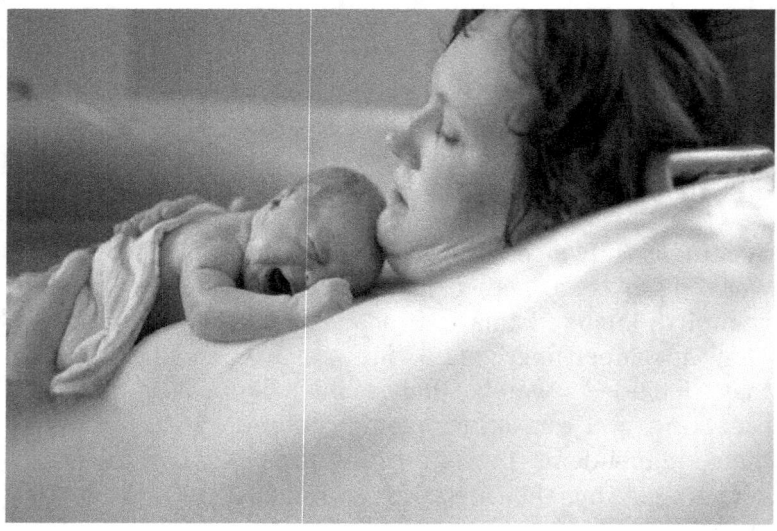

Choosing homebirth requires a deep desire and commitment to do it. Couples and individuals can save money by choosing it, but cost is not a sufficient reason and motivation. The most successful ones are those who trust the natural ability of their body to do the tremendous task at hand. At the same time, they are devoted to doing research about homebirth and will even invest more time and energy in finding the best birth practitioner.

Reassurance and comfort are also reasons why mothers prefer homebirth because usually, the entire family is in attendance during this time. Others find medical assistance an invasion of privacy.

Anyone attending a homebirth is typically called a practicing midwife. However, other homebirth practitioners also include chiropractors, nurses, family practitioners, physician's assistants, and naturopaths.

Water Delivery

Water delivery is one of the most popular natural birth methods used today. Many find it relaxing to give birth in a tub of warm water, usually with a partner or husband in the tub. The water and its buoyancy act as a pain relief and it also reduces pressure and discomfort. It also ensures that the baby does not encounter too much sound and light as it leaves its mother's womb.

However, water delivery is not for everyone. High-risk pregnancies should not go for this option. Women with the following should opt for birth with medical assistance:

- Preterm labor because the baby will most likely need to be put in NICU, or Neonatal Intensive Care Unit.
- Breech baby because it will need Caesarian section.
- Pregnancy complications including Preeclampsia and gestational diabetes
- Diabetes, hypertension, and any other chronic medical conditions.
- Herpes because it easily spreads in water
- Previous Caesarian operation and any delivery or labor difficulties

Lamaze Method

A French Obstetrician, Dr. Ferdinand Lamaze, designed this method. In the USA, this technique has been in use since the 1950s. It comprises of lessons that teaches how pregnant women can increase their ability and confidence to give birth naturally. Before, lessons are focused on techniques to control breathing to cope with labor. Today, a Lamaze course include following:

- 12 hours of lessons but a class should not include more than 12 couples. It is recommended for pregnant women to take the lessons at the beginning of their 7th month of pregnancy.
- 6 birth practices
- Proper breastfeeding and early interaction with baby
- Complications during birth and necessary medical interventions
- How to properly communicate pregnant women's needs with a healthcare team
- The importance of one-on-one professional support
- Tips to help husbands and partners support and encourage their wives during labor
- Natural strategies and relaxation techniques to ease labor pain
- Tips to help husbands, partners, friends, and other family members to be well-informed and become active participants during labor
- Proper normal labor and birth

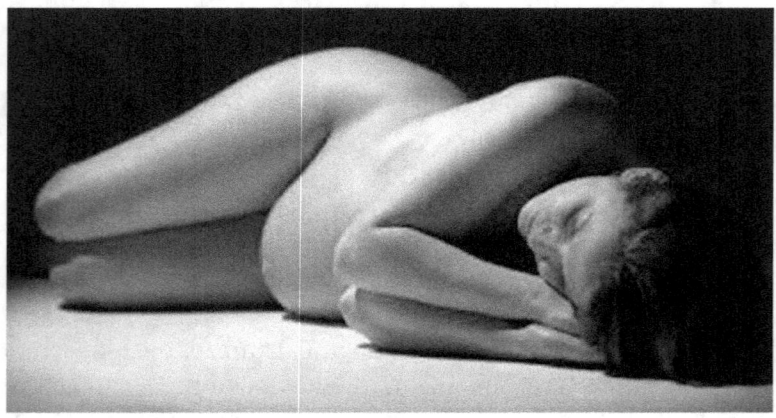

Hypnosis or Hypnobirthing
Dr. Grantly Dick-Read pioneered the use of hypnosis during labor in the 1940s. The Hypnobirthing method aims to bring pregnant women in a total relaxation state. In this state, the female body's muscles can do its job according to the way it was intended. Women who use this method have been

known to experience feeling calmness and lost in a daydream, but still in control.

Hypnobirthing prepares and guides women during childbirth in an extraordinary and peaceful manner. Its program regards the physical and psychological well-being of pregnant women, their birth partners, and newborn babies, whether it is at home or in a birth center. It is also built around a routine that includes positive body toning, proper nutrition, meditation, and visualization. It also teaches a special relaxation and breathing technique for moms-to-be. Most importantly, it encourages mutual respect between the childbirth practitioner and the birthing family in an alternative or a traditional healthcare setting.

The Bradley Method

Also during the 1940s, this natural birth method was designed by Dr. Robert Bradley. Along with the Lamaze Method, it is one of the primary methods of natural birth used in the United States. It is also known as the Husband-coached Childbirth. This method encourages natural childbirth with few or no medications involved. It includes courses that emphasize exercise, nutrition, and techniques for proper relaxation to manage pain. All these lessons teach husbands as well, to assist their wives during labor.

The Alexander Technique

F.M. Alexander is an Australian actor who had chronic Laryngitis which made it difficult for him to perform properly. As a result, the actor developed the Alexander Technique. It involves techniques for proper moving, standing, and sitting with ease, efficiency, and safety. Pregnant women can use this technique during childbirth to release tension in the muscles, to restore the body's proper posture and original poise, and to increase the capacity to breathe.

Through this technique, pregnant women are taught to add simple modifications in their movements to ease lower back pain, shortness of breath, and digestive problems. By the time delivery occurs, they will be able to focus, calm themselves, and breathe better. This prepares them to push and open the cervix better during dilation.

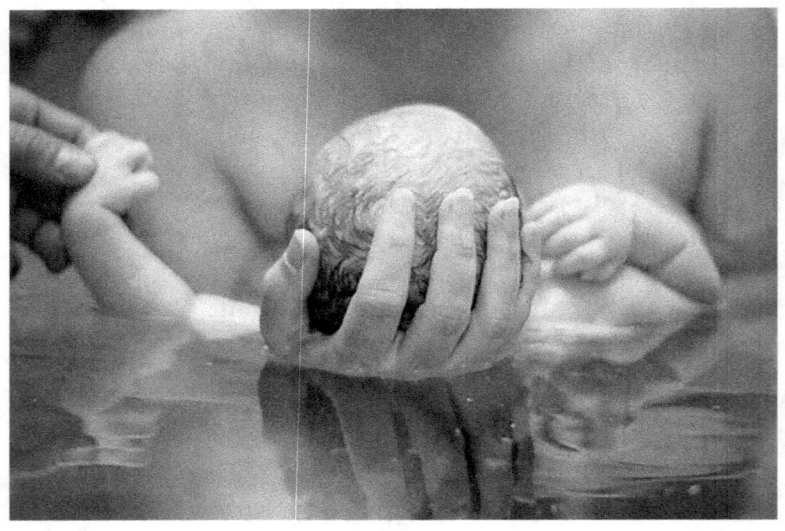

The Leboyer Method

The Leboyer Method, developed by French Obstretician Frederick Leboyer in 1974, aims to minimize the trauma for the baby. This is based on his book, Birth Without Violence.

This method advocates a quiet room, soft voices, low lighting, and sometimes, even soothing music, during childbirth. It discourages tugging, pulling, or rotating the baby's head as it leaves the mother's body. Instead, it allows the mother, baby, and nature to take its course. Afterwards, the baby is immediately, but gently, placed on their mother's stomach where they can be gently massaged and caressed, delaying suctioning and cutting of umbilical cord. Delaying this part of the birthing process enables the baby to breathe on its own without force, instead of spanking them. And then, the baby is dipped slowly in a Leboyer bath, a small tub of warm water, to ease transition from the womb to the outside world by mimicking the weightlessness of the womb.

For soon-to-be mothers, many believe that being brave or becoming a martyr is not the main goal in natural childbirth. It's about treating childbirth as a perfectly natural event and experience. Women find it liberating, rewarding, and empowering.

It doesn't end there. Now it's time to take care of the baby.

About The Author

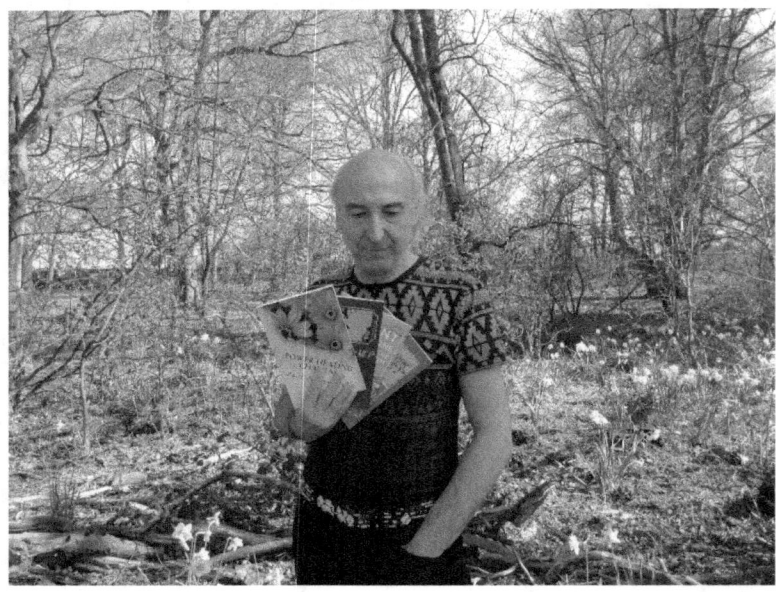

Paul is a senior researcher in Electronic Medicine. Electronic Medicine is a set of modalities and tools that enable the body to be rebalanced, reset. Balancing the meridians does this. He is also a Reiki Master in Usui and Seichim and has been for many years. He is a qi-gong practitioner and practices every day. In his twenties, he was a psychologist in France. He holds a Honors degree from a British University and prepared a Doctorate of Philosophy in metaphysical sciences. He lives in France most of the time. His healing sessions are always free.

OTHER BOOKS BY PAUL ARDENNES

ONE LAST THING...

If you enjoyed this book or found it useful I'd be very grateful if you'd post a short review on Amazon. Your support really does make a difference and I read all the reviews personally so I can get your feedback and make this book even better.

If you'd like to leave a review then all you need to do is click the review link on this book's page on Amazon here:

Thanks again for your support!